I0411964

Master Cleanse

The Ultimate Beginner's Guide for Understanding the Master Cleanse Diet And What You Need to Know

Copyright 2015 by Wade Migan - All rights reserved.

This document is geared towards providing exact and reliable information in regards to the topic and issue covered. The publication is sold with the idea that the publisher is not required to render accounting, officially permitted, or otherwise, qualified services. If advice is necessary, legal or professional, a practiced individual in the profession should be ordered.

In no way is it legal to reproduce, duplicate, or transmit any part of this document in either electronic means or in printed format. Recording of this publication is strictly prohibited and any storage of this document is not allowed unless with written permission from the publisher. All rights reserved.

The information provided herein is stated to be truthful and consistent, in that any liability, in terms of inattention or otherwise, by any usage or abuse of any policies, processes, or directions contained within is the solitary and utter responsibility of the recipient reader. Under no circumstances will any legal responsibility or blame be held against the publisher for any reparation, damages, or monetary loss due to the information herein, either directly or indirectly.

The information herein is offered for informational purposes solely, and is universal as so. The presentation of the information is without contract or any type of guarantee assurance.

The trademarks that are used are without any consent, and the publication of the trademark is without permission or backing by the trademark owner. All trademarks and brands within this book are for clarifying purposes only and are the owned by the owners themselves, not affiliated with this document.

Table Of Contents

Introduction

First off, I really want to thank you for downloading this book. The pages in this book were developed through years of experiences that I have gone through, as well as what has proven to work for others I have talked to and researched. I also want to congratulate you for taking the time to understand the Master Cleanse Diet and possibly leading a healthier lifestyle.

This book contains the origins and fundamental principles of the Master Cleanse and presents the benefits you will get from adhering to it. We will discuss the reasons why it is so popular around the world and why it should not be done for an extended period of time. This short e-book will go through the basics that you need to know before undergoing the cleanse, how to do the cleanse, the ingredients that you'll need, as well as some common mistakes to avoid.

I can guarantee that you will find this book useful if you make sure to implement what you learn in the following pages. The important thing is that you IMPLEMENT what you learn. A change in diet and lifestyle is not conquered overnight but the important thing to remember, is that it is definitely possible for you to make the change over time. What I am giving you is the information you need to get started and the guidelines you will need to make that journey.

I recommend that you take notes while you are reading the book. This will ensure that you get the most out of the information in here. I want you to feel that you made a purchase that is worth your money and I want you to look over the notes of this book even after you've finished reading it. The notes will help you to pinpoint exactly what you need to implement and by writing things down, you will be able to recall specifics and how to handle certain situations when they arise.

Lastly, remember that everything in this book has been compiled through research, my own experiences, as well as the experiences of others, so feel free to question what you have read in this book. I encourage you to do your own research on the things that you want to look deeper into. There are many myths created by supplement and pharmaceutical companies, especially around exotic diets such as the Master Cleanse, mainly because there is profit to be made off of ignorant consumers. You must be aware of what is true and false and that is why I created this book.

The more you understand your own health and body, the better off you'll be. To adopt the Master Cleanse for yourself it will take some preparation and planning on your part, but you can do it! So remember to read with confidence and an open mind!

Chapter 1:

The Basics

The Master Cleanse is a type of fasting regimen that does not permit the intake of food. It substitutes meals with lemonade and tea made with cayenne pepper and maple syrup. The proponents of the Master Cleanse regimen claim that this fasting plan eliminates excess fat and that it detoxifies the body. There is, however, no proven scientific proof that it can eliminate any bodily toxins or that it can achieve any benefits other than temporary weight loss. While having any adverse effects during short-term use is unlikely, it can be harmful if done for a long period of time. The short-term side effects can include dehydration, dizziness, nausea, and fatigue, while long-term side effects can include muscle mass loss.

The Master Cleanse Diet is named after the original book that described it. While the Master Cleanse is usually referred to as a fasting plan, it is really not a complete fast. This is due to the fact that up to 1,300 calories are taken daily in the form of sugar, from the ingredients that make up the Master Cleanse Diet program.

Master Cleanse Origin

It was in 1940 that the Master Cleanse was originally developed in the form of a stomach ulcer cure. It was developed by Stanley Burroughs, an alternative health practitioner. Burroughs' diet book, which was entitled "The Master Cleanser", was presented in 1976. Burroughs by that time was promoting his diet plan, not only as a cure for stomach ulcers, but also for effective weight loss, as well as any other kind of diseases.

Furthermore, Burroughs claimed that his diet plan would result in the correction of all diseases. The public did not readily accept Burroughs' book, as it was hard to decipher. It was in 2004 when Peter Glickman, a huge fan of the diet, published a more comprehensive version of Burroughs' book, entitled "Lose Weight, Have More Energy and Be Happier in 10 Days". Glickman's book was dubbed as the "Lemon Diet" and revived its popularity.

Neither Glickman nor Burroughs was a medical researcher or physician. Burroughs advocated some types of alternative practices aside from the Master Cleanse, such as reflexology, deep massage and life therapy. He was also a practicing vegetarian and nudist. Burroughs was convicted from practicing medicine without a license and for playing a role in the death of a desperate leukemia patient, whom he tried to cure with his alternative practices and master cleansing. Glickman, on the other hand, is a software engineer and a chiropractor who advocated the use of chelation, which was already medically rejected.

Celebrities Who Have Tried the Master Cleanse

Beyonce Knowles and Robin Quivers are among the celebrities who have been reported to have used the Master Cleanse Diet program. It has been reported that Beyonce lost up to 20 pounds in just two weeks in time for her role in the movie, "Dreamgirls". Robin Quivers, who is known as Howard Stern's sidekick, had been quoted by *People Magazine* that she'd heard about the Master Cleanse Diet plan from the popular magician, David Blaine. Quivers was reported to have relied on it for three different occasions, while bringing down her weight from 218 pounds to 145 pounds.

Popular singers Trina and Ashanti were also associated with the diet. Popular actor, Jared Leto, was also reported to have used this diet for his role as John Lennon's killer, Mark David Chapman, reducing his weight up to 60 pounds.

The Benefits of Master Cleanse

There are a lot of beneficial effects of Master Cleanse, both psychological and physical. The Master Cleanse largely enhances your overall health and well-being. It acts to detoxify the body and helps in short-term weight reduction.

Today's modern lifestyle brings about all sorts of toxins into our bodies. We encounter harmful chemicals from processed foods, stress, and pollution. The Master Cleanse Diet, as a detox program, enables your body to purge itself of the numerous dangerous toxins and chemicals.

Junk and processed foods are composed of substances that are hard for the body to digest. This means that byproducts accumulate in the digestive tract and continue to produce toxins into the body after such time, before they are flushed out of the body.

Pollution continuously attacks our body with harmful substances from industrial emissions, car exhausts, and cigarette smoke. Pollution can even trigger health conditions, including asthma and allergies. In the long run, pollution can even lead to respiratory diseases and cancer.

As our body's reaction to stress, it generates substances that are released into the bloodstream. Eventually, these substances accumulate and mutate, resulting in organ failure and heart attacks. Long term exposure to stress can result in a weakened immune system, sexual dysfunction, and skin diseases.

Through a detoxification process, the body flushes out most of these dangerous byproducts from our modern lifestyle and enhances the body's natural abilities to deal with diseases and eliminate toxins.

The following are the reported benefits from doing the Master Cleanse:

Higher levels of energy

Improvement of respiratory diseases such as asthma and allergies

A sense of being calm

Lower blood pressure

Better ability to absorb nutrients, which helps in weight loss and overall health

Lowered acid reflux and ingestion

Reduced wind and gas

Reduced bloating

Fewer instances of headaches

Better concentration and mental clarity

Clearer skin

Improved bowel function

Additionally, the Master Cleanse Diet program is also abundant in Vitamin C. A period of increased intake of Vitamin C, while doing the diet program, can have the following benefits:

Long-term prevention of diseases, such as different types of cancer

Boosting the immune system, which aids the body in naturally fighting off infections and viruses

Promotion of healthy gums

Clearer skin tone and complexion

While the primary objective of the Master Cleanse Diet plan is to detoxify the body, it can also lead to rapid weight loss, as mentioned earlier.

Master Cleanse and Weight Loss

If you strictly follow the instructions of the Master Cleanse Diet program, it will certainly work for weight loss. Any form of fasting will result in a reduction of weight since you are not consuming food, which is dense in calories. In a strict sense, the Master Cleanse Diet regimen is not characterized as a fasting regimen since you will be consuming lemonade containing sugar – around 700 to 1,300 calories worth daily, depending on the number of glasses that you drink.

Therefore, you will experience a calorie deficit every day since the majority of non-overweight individuals require about 1,600 to 2,400 calories daily in order to maintain their ideal weight.

Master Cleanse and Cardiovascular Benefits

There are no known cardiovascular benefits from doing the Master Cleanse Diet regimen. The reduction in weight usually results to heart-health benefits, such as a reduction in harmful LDL cholesterol and lowered blood pressure. There are some clinical studies that have reported constant losing and gaining of weight and showing that being on a long-term diet can stress the heart. This is why it is not recommended to use the Master Cleanse for an extended period of time.

Associated Health Risks

The Master Cleanse program does not reflect any widely-accepted standards for a healthy lifestyle or weight loss. If you consider yourself as healthy, then trying out the program for the first time won't hurt. Although, cycling on and off the diet regimen can set you up for heart and kidney problems, a weakened immune system, long-term weight gain and/or nutrient deficiencies, according to medical research.

Even with sufficient amounts of lemonade taken daily, the herbal laxatives can dehydrate the body and aggravate any kidney or heart problems that you may already have. Irritability, pain, vomiting, nausea, and fatigue are some of the most common side effects. Before trying the Master Cleanse Diet, it would be wise to consult with your doctor to see if you have any pre-existing medical conditions.

Master Cleanse Accepted Dietary Guidelines

Carbohydrates

A sample Master Cleanse menu overshoots the recommended range of 45% to 65%

Protein

A Master Cleanse menu falls short of the suggested range of 10% to 35% of daily calories from protein

Salt

An average American diet is composed of too much salt. The suggested maximum daily amount is 2,300 milligrams. Although if you are older than 51, or suffering from chronic kidney problems, diabetes, or hypertension, the maximum limit is set at 1,500 mg. A sample Master Cleanse menu overshoots with a total of 2,838 milligrams.

Fat

Because you are not allowed to eat solids, you will get far less than the recommended range of 20% to 35% of your daily calorie consumption from fat. A sample Master Cleanse menu just provided 1%. This is one of the key reasons why the diet should not be done for an extended period of time. A long period of time with restricted fats, can lead to damage to your hormone levels.

Vitamin D

Adults who do not get exposed to enough sunlight need to meet the suggested amount of 15 mcg daily with a supplement or food to reduce the likelihood of developing bone fractures. In the Master Cleanse diet plan, Vitamin D is primarily nonexistent. However, you are allowed to take Vitamin D as a daily supplement while doing the diet.

Vitamin B12

It is suggested to get a daily dose of 2.4 micrograms of Vitamin B12 for adults, which is essential for appropriate cell metabolism. The Master Cleanse diet offers none of this nutrient. Vitamin B12 can be supplemented while on the diet.

Calcium

This nutrient is not only important for building and maintaining of the bones but also in allowing the muscles and blood vessels to function properly. The majority of Americans do not get enough calcium through their normal diet. Women, as well as older individuals, must aim to get a daily dose of 1,000 to 1,300 mg. The Master Cleanse Diet regimen only provides 43 mcg of calcium. Calcium can be supplemented while on the diet.

Potassium

Supply of this essential nutrient combats salt's effect of raising blood pressure, reduces loss of bone mass and lowers the risk of developing kidney stones. The recommended daily dose of potassium is 4,700 mg. Unfortunately, the Master Cleanse diet only provides 245 mg. Potassium can be supplemented while on the diet.

<u>Fiber</u>

A daily dose of 22 to 23 grams of fiber in adults will help make you feel full and enhance digestion. The Master Cleanse Diet unfortunately offers negligible doses of fiber.

The Role of Exercise

The Master Cleanse Diet regimen does not mention exercise. In fact, it could even be dangerous to engage in any exhausting forms of exercise when you are eating too few calories. It is wiser to consult with a physician prior to performing an exercise regimen while on the Master Cleanse Diet regimen.

Chapter 2:

How to Do the Master Cleanse

In a nut shell, the Master Cleanse Diet program is this:

The diet plan usually takes around ten days and can last up to forty days.

The only form of nourishment that you will get (without taking vitamins or extra supplements) during the entire diet plan is a special lemonade solution, composed of the Master Cleanse Ingredients, such as water, cayenne pepper, maple syrup, and lemon juice.

An herbal laxative tea should be taken at night. A quart of salt water is consumed during the morning, leading to a number of liquid bowel movements during the day. You will need easy access to a toilet while doing this diet and be sure to stock up on toilet paper.

Over the course of a couple of days, you will have to transition to solid food as you come off the diet. Ideally, you would become a raw food vegetarian, as per the original book of Stanley Burroughs. However, it is not necessary to change to a raw food diet after the diet ends, but be sure to slowly transition back if you decide to go back to eating solid foods.

Master Cleanse Diet Kits

There are several Master Cleanse Diet kits available on the market today. They are available from Maple Valley Syrup, Neera, Coombs, and Peter Glickman. The ingredients for the Master Cleanse Diet are included in these kits, except for the fresh lemons, which you will need to source out locally. There are also some Master Cleanse kits that provide bottled lemon juice.

The Master Cleanse Lemonade

The Master Cleanse lemonade can be prepared within the comfort of your own kitchen. You will just have to prepare and mix the following ingredients:

2 tablespoons of freshly-squeezed lemon juice

Stanley Burroughs suggests using fresh and organic lemons and not bottled lemon juice. Limes may also be used as an alternative. Lemon pulp and zest may also be added. Make sure that the lemons are organic and not treated with pesticides or any artificial coloring.

2 tablespoons of maple syrup

Make sure to use pure maple syrup and not those that are used as pancake syrup. Stanley Burroughs suggests the use of Grade B maple syrup, which is darker and contains more nutrients than Grade A, which may be used as a substitute.

1/10 teaspoon of cayenne pepper

Stanley Burroughs suggests the use of cayenne pepper, although reducing it is permitted if the taste is too harsh for the dieter.

10 ounces of water

Stanley Burroughs suggests using medium hot water, although he also allows the use of cold water.

As a substitute to the lemonade, as promoted by Stanley Burroughs, is the use of 10 ounces of fresh sugarcane juice, although not everyone can gain access to organic and fresh sugar cane juice. Some people who find the taste of maple syrup too harsh, can substitute it with an equal amount of calories derived from organic cane sugar or sugarcane, which can be bought from some health food stores.

The Colon Blaster

Included in the Master Cleanse Diet Plan are the following:

Solution for internal saltwater bathing

This can be prepared by dissolving uniodized sea salt (2 tablespoons) in a quart of lukewarm water.

Herbal Laxative Tea

While Stanley Burroughs is very particular about the kinds and amounts of maple syrup and lemons, with regards to the use of laxatives, he simply recommends, without further elaboration, to go for a reliable brand of laxatives that has been proven to work.

The saltwater bathing solution and herbal laxative tea are the one-two punch that will keep your colon as clean as possible.

To Dos - Before, During, and After the Diet

Day 0 (Day before beginning the diet)

Prior to the diet, you need to select the minimum number of days that you will stay with the fasting program. Buy the ingredients, including sea salt, herbal laxative tea, cayenne pepper, maple syrup, and organic lemons in appropriate amounts to last during the entire duration of your Master Cleanse program. Also, stock up on a sufficient supply of wipes and toilet papers. On the night prior to starting the Master Cleanse Diet Program, take some herbal laxative tea and rest for the night. Remember that for people trying this for the first time, it is best to plan to diet for around 10 days and not longer than 14. After a successful diet, you can try it for a longer period of time on your second go-around, as you will have the experience to go through it.

Day 1 until 10 (or until the duration of your fasting program)

In the morning, drink a quart of saltwater solution before drinking any lemonade. Make sure to stay close to a toilet.

Throughout the day, drink 6 to 12 glasses of the Master Cleanse Lemonade solution. For individuals who are after weight reduction, the recommended amount of lemonade to take is 6 glasses per day. The 12 glasses of lemonade is recommended for those who are mostly interested on the detoxifying effects.

Drink some herbal laxative tea at night.

It is normal to experience weakness, joint pain, vomiting, and dizziness during this period. You may also feel very hungry. Dieters report entering a state of bliss after a number of days, which might be an outcome of the constant elimination of toxins.

Post Diet: Breaking the Fast

When you are done with the diet program, Stanley Burroughs recommends a gentler approach for coming off without drastically upsetting your stomach. Burroughs strongly recommends dieters to follow a raw food vegetarian diet with the following transition process:

Days 1 and 2:

Drink a couple of glasses of orange juice. If there is digestive distress, you may dilute the juice with water.

Day 3:

In the morning, drink orange juice. For lunch, eat raw fruit. For dinner, eat raw salad or fruit.

Day 4:

You may start returning to your normal diet with.

Instead of a vegetarian transition process, you may also opt for an omnivore transition process:

Day 1:

During the entire day, drink several glasses of orange juice. If there is stomach distress, you may dilute the orange juice.

Day 2:

During the morning and afternoon, drink orange juice. For dinner, you may opt to take a homemade vegetable soup.

Day 3:

In the morning, drink orange juice. For lunch, eat vegetable soup with 4 pieces of rye crackers. For dinner, you may eat fresh fruit, salad, or raw vegetables. Do not eat pastries, breads, eggs, fish, or any meat, just yet.

<u>Day 4 and onward</u>:

You may go back to your usual diet, although Stanley Burroughs strongly suggests remaining on the lemonade concoction during breakfast on a permanent basis.

Chapter 3:

Master Cleanse Ingredient Substitutions

Lemons to Limes

The original diet program suggested by Stanley Burroughs recommends the use of freshly-squeezed lemons or freshly-squeezed lime juice. Lemons and limes provide a fresh supply of beneficial enzymes, along with abundant vitamin C and at least 19 other essential vitamins and minerals.

Maple Syrup

Stanley Burroughs suggested the use of Grade B maple syrup due to its availability and calorie and mineral contents for the Master Cleanse fast. However, Burroughs did not mention the use of sugarcane juice as an alternative. Other websites advocating the Master Cleanse Diet suggest the use of agave nectar as an alternative for diabetics who want to follow the program. Agave nectar has low glycemic properties. Burroughs, on the other hand, recommends the use of one tablespoon blackstrap molasses for diabetics as a substitute to the two teaspoons of maple syrup.

Cayenne Pepper

Burroughs pushed for the use of cayenne pepper for his Master Cleanse program. Instead of substituting for it, Glickman suggested that individuals who find it too harsh may reduce the amount of cayenne pepper. Other Master Cleanse Diet websites recommend substituting cayenne pepper with cinnamon for diabetes patients.

The Saltwater Bathing Solution

Burroughs considered the use of a saltwater bathing solution as a superior approach to internal cleansing and advised against the use of colonics as an alternative. Glickman advocates the saltwater flush and recommends altering the volume of salt used, as deemed necessary.

Herbal Laxatives

A couple of substitutes for the Senna Leaf tea include Bentonite and Psyllium. Bentonite is a type of clay that is used to extract the toxins out of the intestine. Psyllium, on the other hand, is a husky fiber which can be mixed in a drink. When you mix Psyllium and Bentonite, they can make a powerhouse laxative. You may use them individually, as well.

Chapter 4:

Pros and Cons

Keeping away from normal solid and junk foods can take the burden off of the kidneys, colon, and liver. Of course, you will instantly feel better by staying away from tobacco, coffee, junk food, and alcohol, without a doubt. However, as with any form of diet, the Master Cleanse Diet plan has its own advocates and critics. The following are some of the pros and cons of the diet program:

The Pros

In the Master Cleanse diet regimen, there is a complete cleansing effect and the colon will be entirely cleaned out by the time the dieter has finished the course of the diet program. The calories delivered by the lemonade drink helps in keeping the electrolytes balanced, unlike a strict fasting plan.

Weight reduction in the Master Cleanse Diet plan is inevitable. The ingredients required for the Master Cleanse Diet regimen are inexpensive to purchase, and they may even be present in your home already. The diet regimen has been reported to provide increased energy levels in many people. People have reported feeling better by engaging in this diet plan, since they have kept away from ingesting toxins in their bodies.

The Cons

Due to protein deprivation, the lean muscle mass in one's body may also be depleted. Fasting is a process characterized by voluntary starvation. It may result in the breakdown of lean muscle mass, which serves to supply energy. This is a survival process of the body that serves to keep an individual alive and maintain normal bodily functions, in the case that they do not get food for an extended period of time. Because of this, the Master Cleanse Diet is not recommended for someone who's top priority is to keep muscle mass, or perform in an activity that requires a high level of strength.

As another con, continuous intake of pure sugar contained in maple syrup can pose a number of dangers. Sugars taken without enough amounts of protein, vitamins and essential minerals will not be able to be metabolized optimally by the body. Also, sugars tend to increase the amount of triglycerides in the blood. Sugars also demineralize bones and teeth. The negligible dose of minerals found in Grade B maple syrup cannot work to offset the harmful effects of all the sugars.

Finally, sugar promotes the development of fungal cells, including candida yeast. Fungal overgrowth in the body can produce mycotoxins that can impair many body parts, including the nervous system and the brain. This condition may lead to digestive disturbances, immune system disorders, headaches, mood disruption, and can be a host for other serious disorders.

The Master Cleanse Diet can lead to the depletion of essential minerals. While the advocates of the diet regimen underscore the fact that suggested Grade B maple syrup is composed of trace amounts of minerals, it can never be sufficient to sustain enough electrolytes such as salt, potassium, magnesium, and calcium found inside the body. Also, sugar metabolism can deplete all the minerals, which negate all the benefits that would be reaped from doing the diet regimen. For instance, insufficient amounts of magnesium in the body can lead to heat arrhythmias and can eventually lead to heart fibrillation.

The Master Cleanse Diet regimen, after being performed for an extended period of time, could lead to the erosion of teeth enamel. Sipping lemonade, an acidic juice, for a period of time can deteriorate some of the enamel of the teeth. Be sure to clean your teeth at least twice a day during the fast.

The nightly intake of an herbal laxative, as suggested by the Master Cleanse Diet regimen, can damage and irritate the lining and nerve endings of the colon. The principle behind the diet plan is to try and keep active bowels while no food is being consumed.

Just as with many other forms of fasting regimens, the Master Cleanse Diet can impair the thyroid glands. This is due to the fact that food deprivation can slow down the thyroid in an effort to save energy. In addition to this, bringing down the metabolic rate also slows down the body's natural capability to detoxify.

The Choice is Yours

In essence, the choice whether to try the Master Cleanse Diet regimen or not, is up to you. If you are seriously considering it, it is wise to consult with a health care provider or other medical professional. You may think that is not important to check with a professional, but doing so will allow you to make sure that your bodily functions are working properly so that you don't suffer from the health issues that were just mentioned. If your blood work doesn't show any signs of severe imbalances, you will probably have a better experience with the diet than someone who has nutrient deficiencies.

If you are a nursing mother or pregnant, never attempt to do any cleansing or fasting program. If you are an athlete looking to perform in a physically strenuous activity, wait until after the activity is over to begin the fasting period. Lastly, if you are taking any medications, do not discontinue them without medical clearance.

Chapter 5:

Common Mistakes to Avoid

Common Mistake - Number 1:

Not Preparing Properly

The Master Cleanse diet instructs individuals to take in only raw food items for four (4) days prior to the cleanse. Many people tend to skip this instruction and just start with the cleansing part right away. Going straight from eating to starvation will most likely distress your body. You can try eating vegetarian meals for one week, then follow with just taking in raw foods for 4 days. This will help in keeping away any side effects. To avoid headaches resulting from caffeine withdrawal, you may also prepare your body by not cutting back more than half a cup of coffee a day.

Common Mistake - Number 2:

Not Drinking Sufficient Lemonade

The Master Cleanse Diet instructs that an individual must completely drink the 64 to 80 ounces of lemonade daily to prevent dehydration. If you find the cayenne pepper is too strong, drink half without and half with, or reduce the amount of cayenne by half. You can slightly alter the recipe, but try sticking with it as closely as possible, for optimal results.

Common Mistake - Number 3:

Replacing Ingredients

The Master Cleanse Diet book says that you are allowed to replace only one ingredient. This is only true for diabetics. Patients suffering from diabetes can do the Master Cleanse diet, although in place of maple syrup, they must use molasses. Organic lemons are very pricey so you can use regular lemons instead, which will work just fine. As mentioned earlier, bottled lemon juice may not work well.

Common Mistake - Number 4:

Not Having a Saltwater Flush or Laxative Daily

Saltwater flushing and/or laxatives are not pleasant. If you find senna pod tea very strong or harsh, you may opt to use gentler laxatives. According to the Master Cleanse diet book, the lemonade tends to loosen up the gunk from the colon and the laxative serves to push it out. There are some who claim that the colon does not need any cleansing, although, if you have ever tried doing this cleanse and saw what comes out after about five days, you may disagree.

Common Mistake - Number 5:

Never Quitting from Caffeine

Caffeine will only take a toll on your kidneys and may just dehydrate you. While on the diet, do not take in any forms of caffeine.

Common Mistake - Number 6:

Failing to Take Days Off From Work

Doing the Master Cleanse Diet is really not possible if you are working most of the day. During the first few days, you will need to have easy access to the toilet for the entire day. If you really need to go to the office, allow at least 90 minutes after taking the saltwater flush or laxatives prior to leaving the house.

Common Mistake - Number 7:

Not Doing the Post Diet

Your body needs to re-adjust to solid foods after the entire 10 days of fasting. The Master Cleanse Diet has a particular 4-day special ending diet. Failing to observe these instructions can lead to severe digestive pain, as your body will try to kick itself back into gear very rapidly.

Common Mistake - Number 8:

Staying on the Master Cleanse Diet for Too Long

Staying on the Master Cleanse Diet for too long can be a serious health hazard. A number of studies suggest that fasting for too long may lead to different side effects such as muscle aches, nausea, and headaches. Long-term fasting may also cause some rare side effects that include having a persistent cold, a drop in blood pressure, and emotional distress.

If you decide to do the Master Cleanse Diet, it is best to do it the way it was originally designed. While in the future you may do an alternative cleansing technique, it is advisable to do it as strictly as possible for the first time. There is a reason for every instruction found in the book, so treat it as such.

Chapter 6:

Some Final Tips

Stanley Borroughs sternly warned against the use of honey in the preparation of the lemonade concoction or the intake of honey at any time. He described honey as "predigested bee vomit", which he considered popular only for gullible health "foodists".

The proponent of the Master Cleanse diet plan also strongly advises against taking any illicit drugs, excess vitamin pills, or any other kind of strange supplements while on the diet plan. Also, you should stay away from cola, tea, coffee, alcohol, and cigarettes while doing the Master Cleanse Diet regimen. Fortunately, most, if not all, of your cravings will entirely disappear after a few days of the regimen. However, Burroughs allows the intake of mint tea or plain water.

According to both Burroughs and Glickman, no other drink or food may be consumed at all.

Aside from being an effective cure for leukemia, ulcers, detoxification, and weight loss, Burroughs promotes the Master Cleanse Diet plan as an alternative baby formula. Burroughs recognizes that mother's milk is still the best, although when not available, he suggested feeding babies with freshly-prepared coconut milk, with the Master Cleanse lemonade concoction given in intervals. However, this needs to be consulted about with a doctor before putting into practice.

Conclusion

I worked hard on creating the best guide for the Master Cleanse that I could. These are all the strategies and information that has worked for me, as well as others that I have talked to and researched. I hope this book was able to help you to get a better understanding of the Master Cleanse Diet, its origins, benefits, and how to do it safely.

The next step is to put down this book (keep it for reference, though) and weigh out the pros and cons of the Master Cleanse Diet regimen to help you decide if you would like to try this diet program.

If you feel like you learned something from this book, please take the time to share your thoughts with me by sending me a message. I would also appreciate it if you left a review on Amazon!

Thank you and good luck in your journey!

www.ingramcontent.com/pod-product-compliance
Lightning Source LLC
Chambersburg PA
CBHW070607290526
45790CB00002B/810